EAT AND GROW RICH

The Top 8 Healthiest Foods You Should Eat to Grow Rich

Michelle Kahneman

Table of Content

Introduction

Getting rich isn't just about investing in the stock market or making money – it's also about living as long as possible. The best way to live longer and healthier is to eat the right foods, ensuring that your body gets the nutrients it needs to stay healthy and ward off diseases such as diabetes, heart disease, cancer, and more. Read on to discover how you can eat your way to wealth by consuming the top 8 healthiest foods you should eat if you want to live longer and enjoy it more!

Avocado

Out of all the healthy foods on this list, avocados are number one for a reason. They're packed with fibre, healthy fats, and essential vitamins and minerals. They're incredibly versatile and can be used in everything from salads to smoothies to dips. We love to keep avocados on hand because they go well with pretty much anything! And if you don't have time to whip up something new, simply slice an avocado onto toast or throw it into a bowl of oatmeal. The possibilities are endless when it comes to avocados! Whether you need a snack, breakfast, lunch, or dinner, avocados will fill you up and leave your stomach feeling full. While we recommend adding avocados to every meal possible (they make everything taste better!), we also recommend leaving some room for these other seven superfoods that deserve just as much attention. Here are our top eight favourite healthiest foods that you should include in your diet: 1) Avocado 2) Spinach 3) Almonds 4) Dark Chocolate 5) Oats 6) Pomegranate 7) Olive Oil 8) Apples. One serving has nearly 20 grams of heart-healthy monounsaturated fat and 14 grams of filling fibre. It also contains more potassium than a banana, so not only does it help reduce blood pressure, but it can also help lower your risk for stroke. But perhaps best of all is that one serving provides almost 50 percent of your daily recommended dose of vitamin K, which is important because studies show that people who consume more vitamin K may reduce bone fracture rates. As far as fats go, they're relatively low in calories and contain no cholesterol!

Pomegranate - Third Paragraph: Believe it or not, there are seeds inside pomegranates! These ruby red gems are easy to peel apart and eat fresh while they're still juicy. If you enjoy tart things, try juicing them before eating them out of hand. If you prefer a sweeter flavor, try dipping them in dark chocolate! Either way, they're great any time of the day and perfect for satisfying cravings when sweet cravings strike.

Pomegranate: Seventh Paragraph This fruit boasts antioxidant, anti-inflammatory, and anti-cancer properties, making it a perfect addition to any healthy lifestyle. Research suggests that pomegranates may protect against diabetes and high blood pressure, two conditions closely linked to cardiovascular disease. So next time you're at the grocery store, don't forget about this tasty fruit! You might want to buy a few extras and tuck them in the fridge. We know they're healthy, but they also happen to be delicious! Pomegranates are in season from October to December and can be found in most grocery stores year-round. What's more, this healthy food tastes like fall! So, whether you're heading home for the holidays or looking for a change of pace, be sure to add this crunchy fruit to your Thanksgiving table.

We know they're healthy, but they also happen to be delicious! Pomegranates are in season from October to December and can be found in most grocery stores year-round. What's more, this healthy food tastes like fall! So, whether you're heading home for the holidays or looking for a change of pace, be sure to add this crunchy fruit to your Thanksgiving table.

Pumpkin Seeds

Not only are pumpkin seeds a good source of protein, magnesium, and zinc, but they also contain antioxidants that can protect your cells from damage. One study even found that eating pumpkin seeds can improve your cholesterol levels and help reduce your risk of heart disease. With all the benefits these little seeds offer, it's easy to see why they list the healthiest foods you should eat!

Açai Berries: If you're looking for something sweet, açai berries have your back. These berries have been known to suppress appetite by slowing digestion and lowering insulin levels (a hormone regulating blood sugar). Açai berries are also rich in antioxidants and vitamins that fight against free radicals in the body, which can cause cancerous cells to grow. In addition, some studies show that eating açai berries can help boost immune system function and lower inflammation throughout the body. To top it off, this fruit is very low in calories, so go ahead and indulge guilt-free!

Coffee

Drinking coffee may be linked to lower rates of depression and anxiety, better cognitive function, improved moods during menopause, or other hormonal changes during pregnancy. A new study has shown that those who drink two cups of coffee daily had fewer strokes than those who drank no more than one cup daily. Another report finds that people who drink at least four cups per day could lower their risk of type 2 diabetes by up to 10%. Coffee drinkers also have an 18% reduced risk of developing kidney stones and a 14% reduced risk of developing dementia. What's not to love about coffee? It tastes great, it's packed with antioxidants, and drinking coffee regularly might lead to weight loss. The beans are healthy, too; just a quarter cup of raw coffee beans packs tons of minerals like potassium, iron, zinc, manganese, copper, and magnesium. Hazelnuts: These nuts pack quite the punch when it comes to nutrition; hazelnuts are loaded with fibre, vitamin E (helps promote healthy skin), folate (important for pregnant women), vitamin B6 (plays important roles in brain development), and many other nutrients that work together to keep your body running smoothly. Plus, they taste amazing! Get ready to dip some raw hazelnuts into dark chocolate, use them as a topping on ice cream sundaes, or enjoy them as part of your favorite breakfast recipe. Tahini: Tahini is made from ground sesame seeds and is high in calcium, vitamin E, selenium, magnesium, and zinc—all important for bone health. This delicious paste can be used in salad dressings, sauces, and soups or simply eaten straight out of the jar. Yum! Chia Seeds: Chia seeds are high in omega-3 fatty acids—the same found in fish oil—that contribute to heart health.

One tablespoon provides 3 grams of plant-based protein and 5 grams of fiber—which aids digestion and helps maintain stable blood sugar levels. These seeds are also a great way to stay hydrated and satisfy your hunger because they expand in the stomach and take up a lot of space. Quinoa: Quinoa is gluten-free, non-GMO, and, most importantly, tasty! Quinoa is one of the few grains that offers complete protein (containing all 9 essential amino acids), making it a perfect choice for vegetarians or vegans. It's also high in magnesium, riboflavin (a vitamin that aids energy production and supports neurological function), and antioxidants. These tiny grains are also fairly light in calorie content—perfect for dieters who need to be mindful of what they put in their bodies!

Beets: Beets are one of the healthiest vegetables you can find.

Cauliflower

This healthy veggie is low in calories but high in fibre and nutrients, making it a great addition to any diet. Plus, research has shown that cauliflower can help boost heart health, improve digestion, and even fight cancer. So, eat up and enjoy! Healthy foods taste good and make you feel good by boosting your immune system and fighting off disease. These are the top 8 most healthful foods to incorporate into your diet: Cauliflower- is a perfect vegetarian option for all you meat lovers. Cauliflower contains vitamin C, lowering inflammation caused by exercise or injury. One study found that people who took 500 milligrams of vitamin C daily were less likely to experience asthma attacks than those who didn't take the supplement. Salmon-These fishies are rich in omega-3 fatty acids, linked to a reduced risk of stroke and improved brain function. Add them to sandwiches, tacos, or salads for an extra protein punch! Chia seeds contain more calcium than milk and just about as much protein as eggs. They're loaded with antioxidants and other essential vitamins like A and E.

What's more? The plant is easy to grow at home--just sprinkle them over yogurt or cereal for an instant breakfast treat! Tofu-Tofu doesn't just have enough protein; it also helps regulate blood sugar levels because it's so low in fat and carbs. It's such a smart choice for weight loss since it fills you up without filling you out. Dark chocolate-It may seem counterintuitive, but dark chocolate is considered one of the healthiest foods on this list. That's because dark chocolate offers protection against stroke and heart attack thanks to its flavonoids called polyphenols, which provide antioxidant benefits and anti-inflammatory properties. Blueberries-This delicious fruit packs tons of polyphenols called anthocyanins that act as powerful antioxidants in our bodies. Blueberries also have incredible anti-inflammatory properties, promoting cardiovascular wellness and improving skin conditions like eczema and psoriasis. They're low in sugar and carbohydrates, meaning blueberries are perfect for people with diabetes and anyone trying to reduce sugar intake. Broccoli-Broccoli is packed with vitamin K, which aids bone strength and prevents osteoporosis. One cup has 34% of your daily requirement of vitamin K. Sweet potatoes-These powerhouses are filled with Vitamin A (beta carotene) that keeps skin healthy and protects eyesight. Just one sweet potato provides 37% of the recommended daily allowance of Vitamin A - try adding it to soup or baked goods like pancakes! Avocado-One avocado provides 20 grams of heart-healthy monounsaturated fats per serving, plus you get 4 grams in each tablespoon of guacamole dip you make yourself. Even better, it has a ton of potassium and vitamin C. Almonds-Almonds is one of the healthiest nuts because they're full of good fats that keep you feeling fuller. They also protect your heart and lower your cholesterol. Almonds are also a good source of protein, especially for vegetarians. Brown rice-Brown rice is full of healthy B vitamins, magnesium, and selenium that are beneficial for your immune system and mental health. Mung beans-Mung beans have plenty of antioxidants and anti-inflammatory properties that make them a perfect food to add to your diet if you want to reduce inflammation in the body or just want to be healthy!

Broccoli

This green veggie is not only low in calories but also high in fibre and vitamins A, C, and K. It's a great food to eat if you're trying to lose weight or maintain a healthy weight. Plus, it's been linked to lower cancer and heart disease rates. The vegetable has even shown promise as an anti-inflammatory agent and can reduce your risk for diabetes. This cruciferous vegetable is one of the best foods for good gut health, so it's essential for digestive system support. If you don't have time to cook the broccoli yourself, purchase some pre-chopped broccoli florets at the grocery store. They make it easy to add this nutrient-rich veggie into your diet with minimal preparation time! In addition to eating broccoli, add cauliflower and cabbage (both cruciferous veggies) to your plate too. Leafy greens like spinach are another nutritious veggie that makes a perfect addition to any meal. Throw them on top of eggs for breakfast or mix them in with pasta dishes for dinner - there are tons of ways you can incorporate these powerhouses into your meals every day! These vegetables will give you extra energy and ward off chronic diseases while boosting your immune system. Garlic: Although garlic isn't known as a low-calorie food, studies show that adding it to your diet could help keep blood pressure levels down. That means garlic may be able to reduce the risk of stroke and coronary artery disease. Garlic contains allicin which is thought to prevent the hardening of the arteries by slowing blood clotting. As a bonus, garlic helps fight infection and promotes bone strength! When buying garlic, always opt for fresh rather than powdered. Mushrooms: Besides being low in calories and carbohydrates, mushrooms contain antioxidants called polyphenols, which may protect against certain cancers, including breast cancer. Mushrooms also contain selenium which boosts the body's natural antioxidant defences. Walnuts: One ounce of walnuts provides nearly two-thirds of the daily value of omega-3 fatty acids, making it a good choice for those who want to live longer or avoid cardiovascular problems. Nuts also provide protein, so they make a satisfying snack with fresh fruit such as apples or bananas. Quinoa: One cup of cooked quinoa offers twice as much protein per serving than brown rice and nearly twice as much fibre! Quinoa is a gluten-free, cholesterol-free whole grain. Adding it to your diet can increase your magnesium, folate, and manganese intake. You'll also get a big dose of protein from just half a cup! All the amino acids in quinoa make it a complete protein source, which benefits vegetarians and meat-eaters alike. Almonds: High in vitamin E and other nutrients like copper, almonds are well worth their cost. An ounce of almonds provides about 18% of the recommended daily vitamin E intake - meaning you'll be less likely to suffer from inflammation or oxidative stress. Just one ounce of almonds packs 7 grams of fibre! Chocolate: Don't write chocolate off as unhealthy just yet! This sweet treat is a good option for those with a sweet tooth and can benefit weight loss. Studies have found that people who ate the most chocolate gained a slimmer waist than those who ate none! The magic ingredient in cocoa beans is an antioxidant called epicatechin which gives dark chocolate its signature taste. Darker chocolates also contain more flavonoids, which have been linked to lower cancer and heart disease rates. This delicious food can be eaten as is or paired with nuts, fruits, or milk to create a decadent dessert or indulgent morning treat!

Eggs

1. Eggs contain all the essential amino acids our bodies need to build muscle and repair tissue.

2. Eggs are an excellent source of choline, which is important for brain health.

3. The yolks contain lutein and zeaxanthin, two important antioxidants for eye health.

4. Eggs contain vitamin D, which is important for bone health.

5. Eggs are a good source of omega-3 fatty acids, which are important for heart health. 6. Eggs are also high in selenium, which helps with immune function and thyroid function.

7. Eggs are low in calories and fat, so they're perfect for people who want to lose weight or lower their cholesterol levels.

8. Eggs have reduced the risk of cardiovascular disease and type 2 diabetes (1). 9. Studies show that eggs may increase levels of HDL (the good cholesterol) while lowering LDL (bad cholesterol) and triglycerides in adults with metabolic syndrome (2). 10. Regarding protein, eggs can't be beaten; one egg contains about six grams of

high-quality protein! 11. Eating more eggs could help you get enough iron if you're not getting enough from other sources (3) since one egg has about one milligram of iron! 12. If you've got a sweet tooth, don't worry - eggs can satisfy your craving! One cupcake has about 100 calories, while an egg contains just 70 calories. 13. So there you have it - the top eight healthiest foods you should eat to grow rich. They won't leave you hungry and will fill your body with everything it needs to live life to its fullest! What are some of your favourite things to eat? Do you agree with this list? Let us know in the comments below! We love hearing from our readers! Below are some responses we've received so far: I always like when articles make sense and back up claims with references. I enjoyed reading this blog post because I learned something new. This post was helpful because I knew nothing about most of these items. The content was interesting and well organized. Keep the feedback coming! We're always excited to hear what you think about our posts. Here's what a few of our readers had to say: I enjoy reading any information that offers alternatives or options for a healthier lifestyle. It's great to see this topic covered in such detail. I love food and feel the same way. Ever since my mom showed me how to cook, I've made my version of pancakes. For instance, instead of using flour, I use oatmeal. And instead of regular milk for the batter, I use almond milk. This healthy alternative is easier on my stomach and tastes delicious too! Cooking breakfast has become one of my favorite things to do now. I've found that changing my diet and cooking meals have greatly helped with my energy levels.

I hope you enjoyed this post! We're always looking for new ideas to share with our readers, so please comment below if you have anything to add! We always appreciate your input. We were surprised to learn that one egg has about six grams of high-quality protein! Who would have thought, right? To provide a little more info, one egg is about 80 calories and provides roughly nine percent of the recommended daily intake for protein.

Chia Seeds

These little seeds are some of the most nutrient-dense foods on the planet. Just one ounce of chia seeds contains 11 grams of fibre, 4 grams of protein, and a host of vitamins and minerals. Chia seeds are also a great source of omega-3 fatty acids, essential for heart health and cognitive function. Add chia seeds to your diet by sprinkling them on top of cereal or oatmeal, mixing them into smoothies, or using them as an egg replacement in recipes. The best part? They have no taste! So, they can be added to anything you eat without changing the flavour. Almonds: Almonds contain vitamin E, magnesium, copper, manganese, riboflavin, and biotin - all-important nutrients that can help maintain skin elasticity and promote hair growth. One serving size of almonds is about 10 nuts and packs 160 calories. Go ahead - enjoy that handful every day! Avocados: Avocados are full of healthy fats that reduce bad cholesterol levels in the blood while increasing good cholesterol levels. They're also rich in carotenoids like lutein and zeaxanthin - two antioxidants that protect eye health from oxidative stress caused by UV light exposure (including computer screens). The kicker? Their creamy texture makes it easy to dress up any dish with a touch of avocado goodness. Spinach: Popeye was onto something when he touted spinach as his power food. It's packed with vitamin K and iron, both crucial for bone strength and immune system health. Even better, spinach has been shown to fight inflammation thanks to its high concentration of chlorophyll - the same stuff that turns plants green!

For breakfast, try having fresh spinach sautéed with mushrooms over toast or eggs. Brussels Sprouts: Cooked properly, these tiny cabbages are delicious! They provide plenty of fiber, folate, and other B vitamins like niacin, thiamine, riboflavin, pantothenic acid, calcium, phosphorus, and potassium. Be sure to buy Brussels sprouts that look bright green and feel heavy for their size. Check out a farmer's market if you can't find them at your local grocery store! Edamame: We highly recommend giving it a shot if you've never tried edamame before. These soybeans are boiled in their pods until tender, then tossed with salt or spices like garlic or ginger before being eaten whole as if they were corn kernels. But what sets edamame apart is their excellent source of plant-based protein and amino acids such as methionine and cysteine, which are key building blocks for muscle repair after exercise. And because they are so low in carbs, you can even indulge in a second helping guilt-free! Sweet Potatoes: The ultimate comfort food, sweet potatoes are loved by everyone. They're packed with vitamin A and beta-carotene - important for maintaining healthy vision and a strong immune system. And did you know those sweet potatoes are also one of the few vegetables that naturally contain significant amounts of vitamin C? The average American only gets about 90% of their daily recommended intake from fruits and vegetables, so it pays to broaden your horizons when picking produce. This is why the most important rule for a healthy lifestyle is to eat the rainbow. There are so many varieties of vegetables and fruits that it can be hard to choose which ones to include in your diet. That's why it helps to list the ones you like and stick with them. You'll also want to pay attention to portion sizes, as some foods contain more calories than others. Remember - this is about balance! We should always take care of our bodies by eating foods that nourish us from the inside out. The last thing you want is for your diet to backfire on you.

Berries

Blueberries, blackberries, raspberries, and strawberries are all rich in antioxidants, which have been linked to lower rates of heart disease and cancer. These little berries are also packed with fibre, vitamins, and minerals. Just a handful of days can give you a boost of energy and help you reach your goals. Make sure to include these delicious fruits on your shopping list. -Strawberries: Are one of the most nutrient-dense fruits because they are low in calories and contain high levels of vitamin C, potassium, and folate. The best part is that they come into season during the summer, so be sure to stock up while they're available!

-Blueberries: As previously mentioned, blueberries are high in antioxidants that protect against heart disease and cancer and boost moods! They contain ample amounts of vitamin C and fibre, which promote weight loss because they make you feel fuller for longer periods. Some studies suggest that eating an apple daily may help prevent age-related cognitive impairment. A study from 2008 found people who ate more apples had higher scores on tests related to mental agility than those who didn't eat apples at all. Add some of these healthy treats to your diet today! Apples, walnuts, green beans, watermelon, grapefruit, celery, and cabbage are all excellent additions to any meal. Studies show that including them in your diet will increase your life expectancy by years or decades, depending on your country. Celery is surprisingly high in sodium (even if it doesn't taste salty), but adding it to any meal will help curb salt cravings throughout the day. Research has shown it helps reduce the risk of developing kidney stones and decrease risk factors for cardiovascular disease too! And don't forget about cabbage; not only does it have great nutritional value, but research has shown that this vegetable can halt tumour growth! Be sure to find ways to sneak some of these superfoods into each meal if possible. For example, add chopped tomatoes and onions to scrambled eggs. Adding veggies like broccoli or carrots to your pasta sauce is another way to incorporate these foods into everyday meals. Try making salsa with tomatillos instead of tomatoes! There are so many different things you can do that won't alter the flavour of your food too much. It's worth a try! What have you got to lose? What would happen if you just kept eating junk food, being lazy, and continuing to grow older? Put down that sugary snack and try something new! Get creative with your cooking, mix these superfoods, and see how long you'll keep that youthful glow. Remember, you're worth it! If you want to improve your health, consider it an investment in yourself if you spend $10 on a gym membership, $1 on a salad, and another $3 on healthier snacks, which adds up to $14. Would you rather spend that money on a weekly McDonald’s habit? Most people would rather spend their money wisely and reap the benefits of a better quality of life.

Nuts

Almonds, cashews, and pistachios are a few healthy nuts you can eat to help you grow rich. Nuts are packed with nutrients like fibre, protein, and healthy fats that can help keep you feeling full and satisfied. They're a great source of antioxidants that can help protect your cells from damage. Walnuts, in particular, contain omega-3 fatty acids, which have been shown to improve brain function and may even slow down aging. What's more, walnuts are loaded with alpha-linolenic acid (ALA), an essential omega-3 fatty acid that helps fight inflammation in the body. It has also been linked to reducing the risk of developing type 2 diabetes and managing weight issues. Other excellent choices include Brazil nuts, almonds, pecans, hazelnuts, macadamia nuts, pistachios, and pumpkin seeds. These offer wonderful nutritional benefits that will help you live a long life while growing rich! So, there you have it! Eight foods that are good for both your health and your bank account.

What do you think? And here is one of our favourite recipes: Arugula salad with garlic chickpeas and sunflower seeds. All you need in this recipe is arugula leaves, red onion slices, olive oil, black pepper, garlic cloves, and roasted sunflower seeds. First, roast the sunflower seeds in a pan on medium heat for about 10 minutes until golden brown. Add minced garlic cloves and cook for another minute until fragrant. Take off the heat and set it aside.

Next, put arugula leaves in a bowl, drizzle with some olive oil, and season with salt, pepper, crushed black peppercorns, crushed red chili flakes, and lemon juice. Finally, top the dish with sunflower seeds and red onion slices before serving it up. Enjoy!
Suppose you want more ideas or to see how other people made their dishes check out these other interesting foods we recently covered. One of my favorites was celery soup, which makes a great meal when served along with avocado toast. Then there's chocolate avocado mousse cake, perfect for those craving something sweet but healthy. Last but not least, who could forget that classic good-good cookie? Yum! There are so many delicious ways to eat healthy while growing rich.

Conclusion

We all know that living a healthy lifestyle takes work. We know we need to eat well, exercise, and stay physically and mentally healthy if we want to be around to see our children grow up, watch our grandchildren play, and keep enjoying life as long as possible. However, many of us let busyness or the monotony of healthy living prevent us from making lasting changes in our daily lives. Many struggles with making a healthy living into more than a fad or trend. Getting fit can seem impossible if you try to take on too much all at once, but breaking it down into smaller, manageable steps makes it easier to stay on track and keep reaching your goals.

www.ingramcontent.com/pod-product-compliance
Lightning Source LLC
LaVergne TN
LVHW052112160826
845678LV00015B/3505

9798840722978